Balancing the Scale

What I Gained While Losing 150 Pounds

By

Tiffini Holmes

Printed in the United States of America

First Printing, 2017

ISBN 978-1545365717

TTWC Publishing
844-367-6968
www.totaltransformationcoaching.com

Dedication

To my parents: Everything I am is because you taught me or gave me the courage to try and learn on my own. Your unconditional love is the safety net that gives me the freedom to jump.

To my trainer: You took a chance on me when others wouldn't. You believed I could even when I doubted. You fought me, for me, and as a result WE won. Your friendship and dedication to me are priceless.

To my friends that are like sisters: You know my best and my worst and you never waiver. THANK YOU!

To God: Only with You is anything I do possible. All I want to do is be in position to introduce others to Your love and Your light. Thank you for entrusting me with this calling.

Foreword

Tiffini Holmes is a Warrior! She just may be the strongest human being that I've ever come in contact with, to date. Ever known anyone that was willing to work hard as possible, learn as much as possible, and do even more to succeed? That's Tiff! With the help of this one Marine guy, (ME) Tiffini used these same skills to lose over 150 lbs., and change her life forever.

When I first met her, she was this beautiful woman, full of life, full of joy, and full of reasons to make a change.

Her previous trainer was a great guy, but couldn't put together the appropriate training program that would complete the process. Looking back, I would like to thank him because he helped spark a flame that burns to this day. A flame that has turned this woman into a machine that thrives off of blood, sweat, and tears.

Our journey would not have been possible, if not for the dedication of Tiffini. We've laughed, cried, fought, and laughed again during our time together as trainer/client. It has ignited a friendship like no other, one that has spawned a boatload of weight loss, a couple of business ventures, and the influence over a growing community of positivity. She has become a complete winner! Part of the crowd that talks less, does more, and won't stop until she has a following that looks to do the same.

During this time as her private fitness trainer, her business partner, and her friend, I've had the honor to work with her as close as possible. I've learned from her, taught her, and influenced her lifestyle for years to come. I can't begin to express the joy I have for Tiffini, and how far she has come. With continuous hard work, dedication, and the will to succeed, the sky is the limit. I look forward to many years of progress, and continued greatness from Coach Tiffini.

-The Fitness Representative, Gabori M. Partee Sr, CFT, PES

Preface: Hear My Heart

I confess. I'm not my favorite subject. I could easily go the rest of my life without ever again mentioning myself or anything I'm doing to anyone. It seems weird to me to talk about things I have done or am trying to do. Yet, as an entrepreneur, I'm obligated to talk about me and by extension my business in order to generate interest and then revenue. But, I still hate it!

A couple years ago I attended a dinner party with a friend. I thought we would go, learn how to cook a new dish, have a good time together, eat, and go home. When we arrived everything was going according to plan. We mingled with the other guests but mostly kept to ourselves. We learned how to make some amazing prosciutto wraps, and were enjoying a very good evening until the switch happened. Our host decided that we shouldn't sit at a table with the person we came with. To switch it up, it was requested that we sit with people we didn't know.

I have no problem talking to or

meeting new people. I LOVE people.

However, I have met so many people

more inclined to introduce their

accomplishments instead of themselves

that I cringe at ever being one of "those

people."

Sigh. I sat at a new table. We

started going around introducing

ourselves, telling whom we came with,

blah, blah, and blah. Things were going

good. Each person at our table was

asked to share one experience they

would like to have accomplished before

the end of the year. I decided to talk

about my desire to run a 5k from start to finish without any walking. Nice, simple, to the point, done, no sweat.

Long story, less long, it wasn't over. During dinner, the conversation came back around. My tablemates each gave their experiences and asked me, AGAIN! So again, I went for simple. I talked about wanting to see my business, *Total Transformation Wellness Coaching*, grow. Quickly, the follow up questions began, prompting me to start talking about how I'd lost 80 pounds at that point. I talked about why my business was so important to me, how I wanted to help other people be well, and that my ultimate goal is to teach the importance of total wellness (mind, body, and spirit) to children so they don't have to struggle to learn it as adults.

To me, my story was nothing special. But from the responses I got, clearly it was quite special. I made numerous contacts and people were really supportive of what I wanted to do.

I realized about halfway into my second response that I had stopped giving standard answers and was truly speaking from my heart.

I love what I do. I know that shows up when I'm working and apparently even when I'm not. I shy away from talking about myself and *Total Transformation Wellness Coaching* (TTWC) because I don't want people to think I am trying to brag or sell them my coaching services. However, by doing that I am cheating people of an opportunity to know me, experience my passion, and perhaps be introduced to a life-changing tool.

I learned a valuable lesson that night. When you speak from the heart that is what people will hear and respond to.

Not only did I generate new business but I also made new acquaintances. The law of attraction is real. I no longer worry about sharing my story and how it will be received. As long as I'm sharing from a good, genuine place, it will be accepted. If it isn't that has nothing to do with me and everything to do with the receiving party.

That story is my disclaimer for this book. This book is not a story about how great I am. This book is my attempt to share my passion and love for health, wellness, and total transformation. My hope is that sharing the lessons I've learned on my weight loss journey will make yours a little easier.

Throughout this book I will share with you my own process of losing weight, and going from 371 pounds to 220 pounds, how I am keeping it off and continuing to lose, and what I gained while losing the weight.

As you read, remember that there is no one-size fits all formula. This book is meant to be a tool for you to use to figure out what is going to work for you. However, you now have a successful framework to begin with and are on the path to reaching your weight loss and transformation goals!

Introduction: Eyesight vs. Vision

"Always have the vision to see the great." ~Tiffini Holmes

As a woman who has been wearing glasses or contacts since age 13, every night I get to experience vision impairment when I remove them. I liken it to what people go through in life when they focus too much on just making it through the day. They look up and while they might have made it through their day, everything else around them is blurry, including their life's vision.

In the everyday hustle and bustle of life it's easy to become nearsighted. When this happens, we often only see what is right in front of us: bills, family drama, unfair treatment on the job, and the list goes on. We become so busy doing "stuff" that we lose sight of living to enjoy life, our hopes and dreams, and the pursuit of those things.

Just like we have to check our eyesight at least once a year to make sure things are as clear as can be, we also have to check our mind's eye to make sure we don't lose sight of the vision that we have for our lives.

Through the years, I've gravitated toward water as a way to keep my mind's eye sharp. I can't swim. I can only tread water in 5 ft. or less (don't judge!) but I love being near water. I developed a love for looking at bodies of water when I went on my first cruise.

Every day I would go up to the

top deck and just look out over all that water and try to imagine what might be on the other side. In my mind, it was always something fabulous. I couldn't wait to get to the next port to see what it would be. Sometimes my imagination was a little too active, but other times it was right on point.

Fortunately, I only live a couple blocks from Lake Michigan. I go to the lake to walk as often as possible or sometimes just to look out over the water and imagine all the possibilities life has to offer. I go to the water to make sure that I exercise my mind's vision muscles. When I go to the water I see that there is more to life than the moment. I see the reality of all my dreams. I see that I still have work to do. I also see hope that makes me willing to go out and do the work. The most important thing I see is NO LIMIT. As far as my eye can see there is nothing but water and sky - no land in sight.

When was the last time you checked your vision? You would be surprised what a new prescription will allow you to see!

As you read, think of this book as one long mind's eye exam. As we peel back each layer together it is going to challenge you to see who you really are and more importantly who you are willing to become.

Ready? Let's go!

Table of Contents

Part II: The Body

PART I: The Mind

Have Faith & Work: The Reality

All the so-called "secrets of success" will not work

unless you do. - Author Unknown

"I believe this is my year. I have faith I'm going to finally lose weight. I trust this time is going to be different." How many times have I, you, we, they, said that only to see nothing change? Or is that just my experience?

Many people talk about losing weight. Talk for one hour and you'll burn approximately 70 calories. On the flip side, if you walk for an hour at a leisurely pace (2.5 mph) you can burn 160-370 calories depending on your weight. Likewise, I am sure you burn calories while thinking about losing weight; however, even actively cleaning the house for an hour (while cleaning up your thinking at the same time) can burn 200 calories.

I say grace before I eat. However, is it realistic to ask for chocolate cake (my favorite) to be nourishing to my body? I believe God turned water to wine but asking Him to make chocolate cake good for me might be taking things a little too far! The point is, I can't, in good faith, talk about living a healthy life if I don't actively work toward it.

Belief alone won't make your weight loss goals happen. For years, I would talk about how things were going to change and I really believed what I said. What I didn't do for so long was ACT on any of the things I said and believed. You now have to put ACTION behind your faith.

The same is true of wishing. Wishing isn't working. Wishing alone doesn't cut it. The wish without the work won't be fruitful.

When I was a child I often wished for something and got it. Side note: I only wished twice a year, for my birthday and Christmas and I always wanted the same things: anything Cabbage Patch related, a bike, or roller skates. Even as a kid when I was squeezing my eyes shut tight and making my wish, I knew I had to also drop hints to my parents so they could make my wishes a reality.

As an adult my wishes are by far less material and much more developmental. This means that an external source can't make it happen for me. I have to work for my wishes. It's my sweat and my food selections that contribute to my weight loss wish. It's my networking, marketing, and professional development that advance my entrepreneurial wish. It's my openness to being in a relationship that edges me closer to my wish for a family.

You get my point, yes?

I wish (insert *your greatest weight loss goal here*).

Now you have to add some work (a lot of work) to bring it to pass.

Are you willing to mix some work into your wish? Are you willing to do the work required to turn your wish into your reality?

Let me give you some Wish Wisdom: I have found that the wishes I wasn't willing to work for were usually too small. But the big ones.... those are the wishes that wake me up at night coming up with new ways to make them happen.

Another important aspect of your weight loss journey that you need to accept upfront is that you will make multiple mistakes along the way, before you reach your goal. Accept this as a reality so that you're not thrown off course when it happens. Often times, what begins as one missed workout or bad meal spirals into weeks of counterproductive behavior, simply because falling off track wasn't anticipated.

I will never forget the first time I fell while working out in the gym. Picture it. I'm 45 minutes into a training session designed specifically to kill my fat (and maybe me too). I'm huffing and puffing and can barely stand up and this man (my trainer) is asking me to do some side shuffles?! Yeah okay! Trying to be a good trainee, I line up, get in position, and start shuffling.

The first couple went okay. The next few were cool, and then it happened. That next shuffle didn't quite work out. I tripped over my foot and it was on. I tried to catch myself but I knew I was going down. I was leaning and stumbling, and stumbling and leaning, and then BAM! The floor and I became one. If you're laughing right now, so was I. It was funny and embarrassing all at the same time.

Fortunately, nothing more than my pride was hurt and not too many people were there to witness it. However, from time to time, my trainer and I still laugh about that and yet another fall I have taken since then although he definitely laughs harder than I do!

That was several years ago and I still remember it. Afterwards, for a while I was really reluctant to do side shuffles again. To this day I don't like doing exercises that require me to be imbalanced, jump forward, or go in reverse, (talk about control issues, right?). But I haven't let the falls stop me. Sometimes I have to take an extra 20 seconds before an exercise to talk myself through the fear before I try it but I get it done.

Life is full of falls (at least mine is).

I fell learning to walk and ride my bike. For years I fell repeatedly when trying to lose weight. I have even fallen for the wrong guy before. The list goes on. But after every fall I got up and had success. I can walk like nobody's business. I have kept off over 100 pounds and slowly but surely I am shedding even more weight. And my selection in men has improved too!

Weight loss success isn't exclusive to me.

Success in anything comes when you get back up. Being disappointed, disgusted, and disheartened when you take a fall is real. But staying down is unacceptable! GET UP!

It's hard but I guarantee it won't get any easier later. If you plan to live in a happy, healthy body you have to work for it now so you can learn how to maintain it later. I have been at it five years and it's still hard sometimes but I have FAITH that if I keep WORKING at it, I will reach my ultimate goal! You can too!

The key is CONSISTENCY. Work, work, work, work, work, in Rihanna's singing voice!

Take Inventory: Get Your Life

"Your life doesn't' get better by chance, it gets better by change." ~Jim Rohn

According to Urbandictionary.com, the term "get your life," made famous by Tamar Braxton, is "an expression one makes when someone makes a comment or does something contrary to what you believe is acceptable."

It's easy to see when others are out of order but let's turn our gaze onto ourselves. Look in the mirror and examine if you need to "get your life." What habits do you need to develop in order to live a more healthy life? What unhealthy habits have you been meaning to take control of but haven't yet?

In order to "get your life" you must:

STOP! Whatever you're doing that is contrary to what you want or should be doing.

START! Taking the steps you can take right now, today, to improve your situation.

CONTINUE! Everything you're doing isn't all bad. Focus on the things that are working and keep it up.

Bottom line: We all need to "get our lives." It's so much easier to look at someone else and see the flaws. However, I don't want to be so busy telling someone to get theirs that I don't get mine.

Grab a piece of paper and take a minute now to decide what habits you need to STOP, START, or CONTINUE. This is the first step toward mapping out your own transformation in progress.

Who Are You?

"Be yourself. Above all, let who you are, what you

are,

what you believe, shine through." John Jakes

In the last chapter I asked you to look in the mirror. Who are you? Who has shaped what you see? How accurate is your vision of yourself?

It's important as you get started on your wellness, weight loss, and transformation journey to know who you are. I mentioned in the introduction, every now and then it's important to check your vision. You have to be sure that your eyes aren't playing tricks on you and the "YOU" you see is really who you are and not someone that others have made you out to be.

If you asked me who I am, I would say: I'm a daughter, sister, aunt, and friend. I'm funny (I think), smart, practical, and outspoken. I'm loyal, determined, and destined for success. I'm Tiffini. I am as common as my name and as unique as its spelling. I'm imperfect, impatient, and independent. I am stubborn! I'm an entrepreneur, writer, coach, mentor, and resolutionist.

Even as early as 6th grade I was selected to be on a committee to listen to student disputes and help them resolve their issues. I am strong. I am sensitive (this was a new discovery for me). I am equipped to handle anything that comes my way. I am a jewel (my mom told me that). Ahhh, but because I know who I am, I also know who I am not.

I'm not a quitter, a liar, or a thief. I'm not fearless (but I am working on that). I am not flawless. I am not mean-spirited. I'm not a "hater." I'm not to be taken lightly. I'm a dreamer and a doer. I am a believer and a worker. I am crazy enough to think that anything we set our minds to do is possible if we are willing to work for it. I am convinced that if you are reading this book, you will be transformed by the end.

So now that you know more about who I am, I will ask you again: who are you?

Knowing who you are, now, is imperative

to your successful transformation process.

You're probably thinking, wait a minute! How can she start out asking me who I am, then shift immediately to talking about changing? I confess. I'm a fan of transformation! So much so that I started a business that is all about change and even included a synonym for change (transformation) in the title. Change is constant. Change is necessary. However, it is rarely easy.

Transformation is an amazing thing. It will cause you to question over and over again who you are. It will also help you realize more clearly than anything else that you are ever evolving, changing, and becoming a better version of you.

Certainly, who you are at your core stays the same. However, you will begin to see early on in the transformation process that you are more fluid than you might think. Who I was when I first started my weight loss transformation and who I am today are so different, and still so similar. Let me explain.

Many of the adjectives I would've used to describe myself before beginning my transformation are still true today; much like the transformation we see when a caterpillar becomes a butterfly. Perhaps all the adjectives that are true today were true then, they were just lying dormant in me, waiting for me to bring them to life. Who I am today was shaped by who I was then.

Transformation also intensifies who you are. If you're strong, transformation makes you stronger. If you're focused it hones your vision even more. The journey of transformation makes you weary sometimes but from that you gain indescribable endurance. Transformation builds off the foundation that already exists. Don't worry if you think your foundation is rocky or unstable. The fact that you have picked up this book and are considering a weight loss transformation of your own indicates that you have a foundation that can sustain change.

However, there has to be an appropriate beginning for lasting change. Meaning you have to start where you are and work your way up to where you want to be. For example, if you are preparing to run a marathon of 26.2 miles you have to first find out if you can at least run one mile. Having this knowledge will allow you to create the appropriate plan to achieve your goal of running a marathon.

Running not your thing, let's talk career. Perhaps you want to be a manager within your company. You need to know what skills good managers possess. You will need to take inventory of the skills you already possess and figure out the skills you will need to acquire. You also need to know your work ethic.

I can't stress this point enough: change is work. Are you willing to do the work to change? This is the first thing you need to know about yourself before you take the steps I go through

in this book. You might be in for a rude

awakening if you go blindly into change without

knowing your predisposition to it.

The Five Stages of Change

"Always remember you are greater than any perceived limitations you have about yourself." ~Tiffini Holmes

There are five stages of change. Most people fluctuate between contemplation, preparation, and action.

Stage 1- Pre-contemplation: you don't think you need to change.

Stage 2- Contemplation: you recognize there may be a problem but you haven't decided it's worth the work to resolve it right now.

Stage 3- Preparation: you're ready to make some changes but you haven't started yet.

Stage 4- Action: you're currently engaged in making changes.

Stage 5- Maintenance: you have completed the change and you are maintaining the new lifestyle.

It's important to know what stage of change you're in so you aren't discouraged by your behavior. If you're in the contemplation stage you're supposed to be procrastinating!

My focus is to get you to the Action and Maintenance stage. While that is the focal point, it is imperative to not skip any of the steps. It's going to be difficult to act if you skip the preparation stage.

Stop Doubting Your Ability, You Qualify

"If you have health and happiness, you have all you need, and the capacity to go after all your wants."

~Tiffini Holmes

It's natural during your weight loss transformation to doubt your ability.

My first thoughts when I started my weight loss transformation journey were: "I can't lose 200 pounds! I can barely lose 20 and even those somehow always creep back. I don't have a clue about working out, nutrition, or anything health related. Everything I know is a fad diet or comes from a magazine's "half their size" issue.

Basically, I didn't feel "qualified" to embark on this type of journey.

The word "qualify" or some variation of it comes up often in life. Whether you're applying for a job or a loan, getting a certification, gaining access to certain social clubs, or even giving advice, people want to know what your qualifications are. Sometimes we question our qualifications or allow our apparent lack thereof to limit us. Thoughts like, "What qualifies me to do this," or "I'm sure someone more qualified than me would be better at or for it."

Qualified is defined as being competent, capable, or fit for a given purpose. Another definition is being eligible, able to meet a requirement. Based on the first definition, I would say we all meet the qualification for achieving any goal we set out to reach. If our goal is to be our best and healthiest selves, we are fit for it because we are capable and have access to all the tools we need. Therefore, we are qualified. Further, we are eligible (the 2nd definition) because the only requirement necessary to be able to pursue our best is to be alive. If you're reading this, you are definitely alive!

That being said, I just proved that we all qualify and have the ability to accomplish our goals. The underlying message, easily missed, is you don't have to have all the qualifications right now. You just need the ability to obtain them. Now armed with that knowledge, we are tasked with the responsibility of beginning.

Being your best self is a much more individualistic concept. In general, I would say it is striving to live at your highest potential. You're working toward being and giving your best in every area of your life: personal, professional, and community. It doesn't mean everything is perfect but you rest easy most nights knowing that life is good and if you keep living, it gets even better. Whatever needs to be in place to get you to that point in your life is your GREATNESS.

All too often, we don't get to our best or our individual greatness because we qualify (which in this case means to restrict or lessen) our abilities. Well, we can no longer afford to do that. It has been established on this day that we are qualified. Greatness is our God-given birthright.

Understand that you are in control over the decisions you make and don't make every single day. For example, knowing that you need to lose weight but avoiding the gym, means you're INVITING the fat to stay permanently affixed to your hips.

I was working out one evening, not feeling it at all, when I got a message from a friend in the area asking me to meet up. The only reason I saw the message was because I was quitting my work out early. Be that as it may, I took the message as a sign that I needed to complete my workout by jogging over to her location. So I began doing my infamous walk/trot/jog-ish thing.

Huffing and puffing, I meet up with her and we talk (well mostly I complain about being tired, sweaty, not feeling the workout, and how I wish I could just get to maintenance mode already).

My friend to the end listened to me for a while. Then she began to tell me how well I've done and to be patient and stick with it. I listen. I knew she was right but all I kept thinking was: for as hard as I'm working, my butt is still too big and my thighs are still too thick. Woe is me. Instead of going back and forth, she decided to take me on a trip down memory lane. We attended a wedding in Jamaica years prior and she had photos to prove it.

She pulled out her phone and pulled up a picture of us from that trip.

"Here! Remember this? This is what you used to look like. This is where you've already come from and look at you now."

Light bulb!

I was easily 75 pounds lighter than I was when I first started my weight loss transformation journey. Looking back at the woman in the picture, I didn't even remember being that big. Looking back helped me see the progress I had made up to that point and where I wanted to be in the end. That was her point! Sometimes you have to look back and remember how far you've come in order to gain perspective on the leg of the journey that remains.

In the midst of that flashback I found an extra burst of encouragement that I needed to keep going. Yes, my butt is still big and my thighs are still thick but they were bigger and thicker before I started. I am doing the work and can now see the results. I just needed a quick reminder of progress made to help me stick to it.

The occasional glance back serves as motivation. It allows you to see how far you have come, the stumbling blocks you avoided, and it gives you a boost of confidence to go on.

The moral of the story: take a look back.

See how far you have come, celebrate every hurdle you've jumped, and every roadblock you've averted. Now look ahead. You're going to make it to your finish line. You got this!

Disciplined Habits Over Time: The Understanding

"Furious activity is no substitute for understanding." H.H. Williams

I was overweight from about the age of 10. However, things definitely got worse as an adult when I was pursuing an advanced degree, working a full time job, dating, having a social life, and doing everything but taking care of myself. I was spending money on travel, eating out, clothes, you name it, and it was nothing to me. I think back and wonder. When did my priorities get so far off track?

I actually thought I was taking care of myself.

After all, I made sure to get my hair done every week; I got mani and pedis every two weeks, and a massage once a month. I was working hard and playing hard. That's what life's all about, right?

Wrong! Honestly, I never had the traditional ailments that come with being overweight. Every time I went to the doctor she would be shocked that my overall health results were so great. However, she knew and I assumed carrying so much excess weight was not good and would eventually catch up to me. So, I decided before that happened, to invest in myself.

The first thing I did was got a gym membership (AND USED IT!). Then I realized beyond walking on the treadmill I didn't know what I was doing in the gym, so I got a trainer. Next, I started investing in what I put in my body. This is not as costly as most people think. Once you learn what to shop for and where to find it, healthy eating is affordable and tasty too!

Education is great. Career advancement is great. SHOPPING is great. Heck, if sitting on the couch watching TV is your thing, that's great too! And there is absolutely nothing wrong with pursuing those things wholeheartedly.

However, NOTHING is more important than your health! Therefore, the pursuit of great health should always be a priority. The next time you find yourself thinking about how much it costs to be healthy, consider the cost of being ill and then spend wisely!

I can't tell you how many times friends have rolled their eyes when I have had to cancel or change plans so I could get in a workout. They sometimes look at me crazy when I tell them I pay for a personal trainer, a gym membership, fresh produce every week, and all the other things that go with this lifestyle of health and fitness, including cute workout clothes with matching gym shoes. My philosophy is: If I have to sweat and look a mess, at least I'm coordinated.

Weight loss success takes discipline and a change in lifestyle habits. It also takes a measure of selfishness and thick skin. Friends, family, coworkers won't always readily accept your choices. The key is to do what's best for you anyway! Knowing what's going to work for you and then doing it consistently is going to put you on the road to weight loss success and keep you there.

Don't look at your life one more day and wonder why things are the way they are.

Begin practicing living the life you aspire to, today.

Say Yes to Snacks

"Pack snacks so you don't have to pack

Spanx." Tiffini Holmes

I'm always packing a bag and heading somewhere. Some days I feel like I live out of a suitcase. I travel locally to see clients for work. I travel to visit friends that have chosen to live all over the country. I also travel to fulfill my need to see as much of the world as possible. I'm so used to it, I have a mental checklist of must-haves that runs on automatic: clothes, glasses, toiletries, iPad, cell phone, chargers, headscarf, snacks, insurance card... Wait, snacks make the list? ABSOLUTELY!

I eat 5-6 times a day. On more than one

occasion for one reason or another I have missed one of those meals and it didn't make me or the people around me happy. Packing snacks minimizes the risk of me using a missed meal as an excuse to go rogue and hit up someone's drive-thru. I take snacks everywhere I go to make sure that doesn't happen. I am like a mom with a toddler. There is a snack survival bag within arm's reach at any given time.

I learned the snack bag survival lesson the hard way. At my previous employer, every week featured 'Fat Tuesday' in the office and I forgot my food bag that day. It was the day I was introduced to a Paczki. Paczki's are similar to doughnuts. They're filled with a variety of sweet goodness. I tried to resist but because I had no alternatives and I was starving, I had 2 Paczki's that day. That was probably close to 1000 calories of sugar, fat, and nothing good for me. Since then, I never leave home without my food bag and snacks already prepared and ready to go.

My travel snack essentials: apples, almonds, protein shakes, and Skinny Pop popcorn.

My friends laugh because I have an early curfew on Sundays so I can prepare my meals for the week on Sunday night. I prep, cook, and pack as many meals as possible so I can grab and go all week. I often leave home by 6 am and don't come back until 6 pm. To minimize stopping for fast food or raiding the vending machines, I take food with me.

The same rules apply for traveling out of the city.

When traveling for work or pleasure you can't always run out to get 5-6 small meals every 3 hours, your restaurant options are limited, and you aren't cooking, so chances are that even ordering vegetables will increase your normal caloric intake. Therefore, it becomes imperative to control your snacking as much as possible and be proactive about what you order at restaurants.

Here are some tips for ordering meals at restaurants:

- Ask questions: ask if veggies are steamed or sautéed in butter.

- Get everything on the side: salad dressing, sauces, and toppings can pack a ton of calories so get them separate so you can control how much of them you eat.

- Be creative: you may have to piece together a meal from several menu options, most restaurants will accommodate if you ask nicely.

- Leave room: not for dessert either! Most serving sizes are too much to eat in one sitting. Don't stuff yourself in the name of getting your money's worth.

- Remember your goal: don't undo all the hard work you've put in day in and day out at home by making bad food choices while away.

"By failing to prepare, you are preparing to fail."

-Ben Franklin

Hold Yourself Accountable

"Without personal accountability we cannot grow nor can we ever improve ourselves." ~Unknown

As a wellness coach I am also an accountability partner. I can motivate. I can guide. I can encourage. The one thing I CANNOT do is complete the job for you.

I can go to the gym and sweat it out every day and that will not change your weight the next time you step on the scale. I can shop the perimeter of the grocery store all day long and that won't change what's in your cart if you choose to go down the cookie and chips aisle.

Bottom line, there is no external force greater than your inner ability. When you decide to be answerable for your choices, be accountable for your actions, and take responsibility for making your goals a reality, no matter what anyone else does to help or hinder, you will be unstoppable!

Don't get me wrong, having support from someone else is always better, but it's not necessary and realistically it's not always going to be available. You must be ready, willing, and able to give yourself a pep talk when you need cheer for your own victories, and force yourself to do what needs to be done.

YOU are the key. I often say, "my weight, my worry. Only I carry it, only I can shed it."

During a conversation with a friend one

day, I was using what I perceived as a lack of support as an excuse for why I wasn't doing something that I was fully capable of doing on my own. My friend looked me in the eye and emphatically said, "I don't owe you anything." It's funny that I remember the intensity of the conversation and how taken aback I was when he said it. However, neither of us can recall the situation that predicated the conversation.

As someone who is pretty independent most of the time and who tries to ask people for very little, my feelings were definitely hurt. However, it got me thinking. I could argue what is owed to me by others in the name of friendship, human decency, and other obligatory facts but after I took the emotion out of it I concluded, regardless of what anyone else does or does not owe me, I owe myself!

Almost every day I have someone ask about going to the gym with me. They say it's so hard going alone and if they just had someone to go with them they could be more consistent. I agree it is much easier to workout with someone else and so I try to never turn anyone down that wants to join me.

So off we go to the gym. However, the minute I have to travel for work and can't go with them to the gym, they fall off. Who's accountable for that? Me? Nope, it's definitely them. The lesson my friend taught me, and yes we are still friends to this day is: the only person that is obligated to show up for me is ME!

Here are some tips and ways to become more accountable to you:

- Recognize your power: Start where you are and learn as you go. You may not have all the answers but you know where you are isn't where you're meant to stay.

- Love yourself: When you love someone there is very little that you wouldn't do for them. When you love yourself, the same rule should apply.

- Set expectations: It's easy to set expectations for others and let them know when they don't follow through. Do the same for yourself.

- No excuses: Don't justify subpar

dedication to yourself with excuses.

Accept it for what it is and make changes.

Our motto (because you now share it with me): I am responsible for MYSELF and my choices. I have to stay focused on becoming a better ME!

Accountability Exercise: What is the plan?

What are the little goals/milestones to the big goal?

1.
2.
3.
4.

What needs to happen?

1.
2.
3.
4.

What steps need to be completed to make it happen?

1.	
2.	
3.	
4.	

What is the frequency?

1.	
2.	
3.	
4.	

The Decision

"A real decision is measured by the fact that you've taken a new action." Tony Robbins

So how did I go from 371 pounds to 210 pounds?

I made a decision. That decision was to take control of my health and lose 200 pounds.

That is a HUGE decision to make when you have had membership after membership, made many unsuccessful attempts in the past, and have no clue what to do now because let's face it, losing 2 pounds can be challenging so 200 seems impossible.

However, I told you I was stubborn, right? Well, when you make big decisions you have to be stubborn, too stubborn to fail. Stubborn enough to take the first step and stubborn enough to keep going!

I will start next week. As soon as I get all the junk out of the house, I will start. When I finish these other things (that I'm not really working on) I will start. I need to do some more research, and then I will start. I know I need to do something. It's not that bad right now, so I'll start working on it when it gets worse.

Do any of the above excuses to prolong your start sound familiar? Have you said or thought these things or something similar?

I have! And guess what? Next week never comes. Those "other things" don't ever get completed.

I get it. I really do. We mean them when we say them. We believe getting beyond these "things" will make whatever we are trying to start easier to attain. I mean, how can you start a "diet" on a Friday? And with junk food in the house? No way! Surely if I wait until Monday and eat this last bag of chips I will be more successful when I try to lose weight right?

WRONG!

The reality is the longer it takes us to start the longer it will take us to finish. Moreover, if we never get started, we will never finish.

The perfect place to start is HERE and the perfect time is NOW! I consider it the difference in running a sprint vs. a marathon. Sprinters have to get down in the blocks, they get into the set position, they wait for the gun, then they go all out for a short period and it's over.

Marathon runners line up somewhere at the start line and then take off. They pace themselves, make adjustments along the way, go the distance, and finish strong.

Have you ever seen a marathon route after the race is over? There are cups everywhere, sometimes sweatshirts, hats, and other trash that the runners have shed along the way.

Marathon running is a parallel for life. Line up at the starting line and go, just as you are, right HERE right NOW. When you need to

get rid of "things" get rid of them as you go.
When you need to pick something up, get it
along the way.

"Things" will never be perfect and if we
wait for perfection we will never get anything
done. So the next time you decide to start
something and you contemplate the best time to
do it, know that the only time is HERE and
NOW!

The Road Less Traveled

"It's okay to be scared. Being scared means you're

about to do something really, really brave."

~Mandy Hale

When I first decided I was going to lose weight I had no idea what I was getting myself into. I thought I would start working out and eating better and the weight would just disappear. Well, it's that easy and that HARD!

The equation is simple but the application is tough. The process doesn't consist of simply working out and eating right for a day, a week, a month, or a year. It is a lifetime thing. Not only is it a lifetime thing but you also have to modify the plan over and over again so your body keeps responding. You have to do it when no one else is doing it and when you don't feel like doing it.

During the spring and summer months, at least three days a week, I walk, trot, and/or jog the same two trails. I know where every dip, crack, and bump is on both. I know when the trail will be the most crowded and when it will be virtually empty. I have landmarks where I slow down and points where I push it. Sometimes I switch things up by alternating the days I walk on each trail but at the end of the day they are still the same two paths.

They are my comfort zone. I feel safe on those two trails. I'm working out, I'm sweating, and I'm dedicating one hour to my wellness. I'm on the right path, right?

WRONG!

One morning I ended up on another trail. I didn't know the terrain. I didn't have my normal landmarks to go by, and I was being pushed to do more than my normal pace. I was so far out of my comfort zone. I didn't like it one bit! But I survived and learned a couple lessons along the way.

There is no challenge in the comfort zone. You know the territory of the familiar path and you've travelled it so much that you know you can do it. There's no risk of failure (this might be a pride issue; or is that just me?).

The only way to get over it is to get out of it. It

might be uncomfortable leaving the safety net of your comfort zone but the reality is, there will be times when we are forced out. The best way to prepare for that is to get out on our own. Change it up, take risks, and get comfortable being in uncomfortable places.

I love my two paths. They're pretty, peaceful, and comfortable. My two paths are also limiting, too easy, and no longer an option.

I wanna grow so I gotta go.

I have to stay out of my comfort zone. What I want for my life isn't there. That is true for most of us. I'm committing to taking new paths. Will you join me? Will you decide to leave your comfort zone and do something amazing?

Check Your Will

"Never hope more than you work."

~Rita Mae Brown

We live in a society where everyone wants to say and do whatever he or she likes but then become sensitive when something is said or done to him or her in return. As adults, we know right from wrong when it comes to what we consume, what we spend, how we live, and how we treat others and ourselves.

We may not know the best things to do, but we definitely know what NOT to do.

However, every day we make decisions that undermine what we say we want for ourselves. Then if someone has the audacity to mention it to us (directly or indirectly) we are quick to take offense.

Several years ago on social media a mom with a great body posted a picture of herself in a sports bra and shorts with her 3 kids and asked, "What's your excuse?" She was making the point that she was a mom and had some of the same challenges many moms face but still found a way to stay in shape. That poor woman caught all kinds of hell. The way she presented the message was less than stellar; however the message itself was accurate. She was checking people and they didn't like it.

In my experience I've found I'm the only person who can truly check me. Other people can inspire me, challenge me, critique me, dare me, and motivate me to change. But it is only when I look at myself, dissect my behaviors, weigh my actions, and check myself that I then begin to make any changes.

If we say we don't need nor want anyone to check us then we need to do a better job of checking ourselves. When something about us needs to be improved, we know it. The next step is to do something about it. Should others stop checking us though? No. Sometimes the only way we take notice of needed changes is for someone else to point them out. But to answer the question, "Who gon check me, Boo?" the answer is: ME!!!! I will check me to change me!

When we decide what we will and won't

do, those decisions then shape us mind, body, and spirit. If we really want different results then we must be willing to make different decisions. I truly believe most people WANT to make changes but somewhere along the way they lose the WILL to make change. So, how do we get it back?

Here are my tips:

Be Real: Very few good things in life come free or easy. We have to work to pay for vacations and other luxuries we enjoy. Most of us had to study to get good grades in school. If you know a thing about love you know it takes a lot of W O R K to stay in a relationship. Why then believe that it should be any less work to start a business, lose weight, or live a more positive lifestyle? Know that to achieve any goal or resolution it will take work. Be willing to do the work in order to get the results.

Remember The Payout Is Greater Than The Payment: Basically the work is worth it. If you hate going to your job every day, if you dread going to the doctor because you know they're going to check your blood pressure and cholesterol and it's still out of control, if you hate coming home because the entire house is in disarray how can you not change that? Yes, changing it will be exhausting, it may not go as fast as you like but in the end you will be better off than you are now. Just like with a 401k, invest now so you can retire later. Initially, the sacrifice may seem like a lot but with consistency it will become a habit with an amazing payout.

No Choice/No Excuse: Technically, taking care of yourself and making sure you are living your life to maximize your happiness is optional. The choices you make to work out or not, to eat better or not, to stay in a dead end job or not all impact your level of happiness. Stop making excuses and giving yourself the choice to be less than your best. Tell yourself your only option is to be a better you tomorrow than you are today. Then don't allow yourself any excuses to take a day off from making that statement true. Quitting, failing, and giving up are not options and should no longer be a part of your vocabulary.

Every Day Counts: It's so easy to take a day off and think it doesn't matter. But it's even easier for one day to slide into two days, then a week, month, or a whole season. In the beginning it's all about establishing better habits. Once something becomes a part of your routine then you can think about taking days off. Every day you should be doing something toward your goal. Treat your new start like a new job. In the first 90 days, no days off!

You Matter: You can like every motivating status you read on Facebook. You can say you're going to start to improve but until you get up and get active you won't see a single improvement. Outside motivators can only do so much. It will be your sweat, your tears, and your work ethic that guarantees your success.

So pack your bags because it's moving day. You're moving from the dead-end, Want To Ave. over to Will Street.

You WILL exceed your goals.

You WILL keep going no matter what.

You WILL win. IF…you DECIDE to do the work!

The pictures we see on social media and in magazine issues dedicated to amazing before and after weight loss transformations, show everyone smiling in the end but what about the in-between? That "dash" makes all the difference. Weight loss isn't pretty, easy, or any other awesome adjective. It is work. It is a mental, physical, and emotional battle. But it is worth it! Your success only comes when you will your way to success each and every day.

Will Exercise: Target Practice

Got your goal? Great! What is it?

_____

Do you have what you need to hit your target? If
so list them. These arrows are the tools that you
can use to reach your goal.

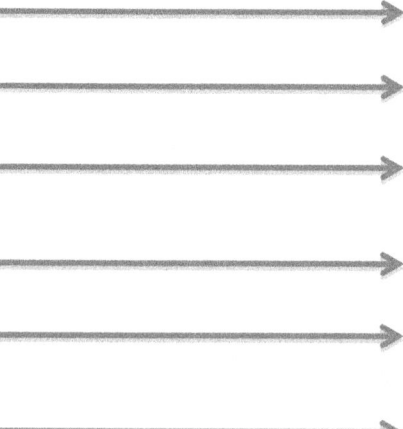

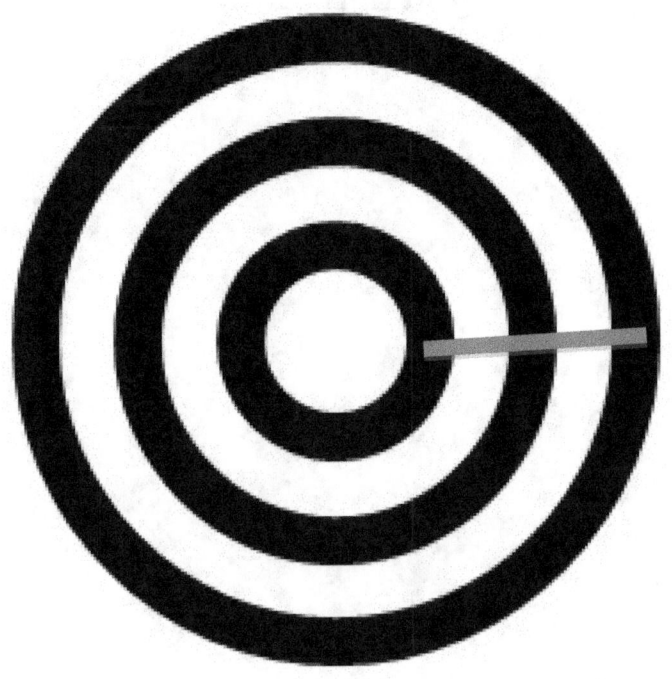

What do you need that you don't have? These incomplete arrows are the tools you have to acquire.

Part II: The Body

The Contract

"Commitment is what transforms a promise

into reality." ~Abraham Lincoln

"How did you successfully lose 150

pounds?" This is the question I'm asked again

and again.

My answer in short is: I decided I wanted

to lose weight. I told myself and my family that I

was going to do it. I came up with a plan of

action where my first goal was to walk up the

flight of stairs from my garage to my house

without getting winded. I made up my mind

that there was nothing but death that could stop

me and I went out and started working on it.

As you see the first step was the decision.

The second step was I made a

commitment to myself and did not leave any room for retreat. You now know what it takes, you know who you are, you have an understanding of how to prepare for, execute, and achieve your weight loss goals. The heavy lifting that starts with your mental attitude and ideas around weight loss and what it takes to be successful, we've gotten through. You now know the potential success and pitfalls ahead. Are you still committed to doing it anyway? Are you ready to get started working on your body? Yes?

Great! Then you need a contract.

This contract is part eviction notice, part goal acceptance.

Date: _____

Bad Habit(s) Name(s):

_____

_____

Last Known Residence (mind, body, spirit):

_____

_____

(Insert your name) you are hereby being notified

to vacate the premises of

_____named above located within

_____.

The reasons for eviction are:

_____

_____

_____

_____

You are required to vacate the premises within 30 days from the date of issuance of this notice. Failure to do this is not an option as you are not a legal resident of my mind, body, or spirit, you are not adding value, and as such you are a guest who has overstayed your welcome and are now officially uninvited.

Basically, you are trespassing in my life and that is unacceptable!

Thank you in advance for your swift and permanent exit.

In exchange for the complete and immediate removal of the above mentioned bad habit(s) I will: (Do what)

_____

_____

(When)

_____

_____

(How often)

_____

_____

(How much)

_____

_____

Print Your Name:

_____

Signature: _____

Date: _____

Invitation Denied

"What you allow is what will continue."

~Unknown

Many major life events such as birthdays, baptisms, weddings, graduations, and even divorces are celebrated by extending invitations to a party or ceremony of some kind. In addition to these major life events, we extend and receive invitations every single day.

Whether it is the look you send to a handsome, young gent inviting him to come over and speak to you (if you're single of course), or a friend invites you to like a page on Facebook (if you haven't liked mine yet www.facebook.com/ttwcoach). Invitations are always going out. They indicate who and what we want to come into our space. Invitations set a standard for appropriate behavior and dress. They often include direction on what to bring.

Let's take it one step further; beyond these formal invitations to events, every person and/or thing in our life is there by invitation only!

Say what? Say word.

Yep, we always have the option to invite people and things, in and out of our lives.

Now I know you might be like, "How do I un-invite my boss, in-laws, baby momma from my life?" Let me tell you how. You may not be able to remove their physical presence but you can remove their negative impact in your life.

The key is to recognize your power. Most people are not ignorant to the effect they have on you. Some people will push your buttons on purpose. How long will you continue to react to the same things in the same way? Your allowing it is an INVITATION for the behavior to continue.

If your boss is a nuisance, diffuse his or her power by not expecting the person to change but by changing your reaction to them. You can also start looking for a new job. You can report them to the next level of authority. You can just come to an understanding that they're moody before 10 am and stay clear until 10:30 am. You can choose to not take their behavior personal.

For the in-laws, talk to them about their issues, if they can't see it, limit your interaction or learn to tolerate it. It may seem oversimplified but what would you rather do? Be miserable or learn to endure?

How do these invitations relate to weight loss? We invite extra calories to invade our hips and thighs (or wherever your problems areas are) each time we make unhealthy eating choices. Additionally, we invite stagnation in every time we allow doubt or complacency to stop us from working on self-improvement.

Begin to look at the invitations you are extending to people both actively and passively. What healthy habits do you need to invite into your life? What bad habits do you need to invite out? Whose invitation needs to be revoked and who needs to be let in? You are an invaluable gift. Invitations to your life should be exclusive and include only things that will enhance you, not drain or detract from you.

The Beginning

"He has half the deed done who has made a beginning." Oliver Wendell Holmes

You have made the commitment to lose weight, now it's time to get to work on it. Remember that a contract is a legal binding agreement and that there is no breaking it. You are in this until you reach the goal you set out in the last chapter. To help you take this a step further, let's work together to get rid of your "buts," before working on your physical butt!

There are silent "buts" that block out your motivation and others that flow freely. Here are some common spoken **BUTs:**

- I'm too busy to cook and workout

- The cost of fruits and vegetables are too high.

- No one wanted to workout with me.

- I can't do it by myself.

Here are some common unspoken **BUTs:**

- I'm scared.

- I can't do it.

- It's embarrassing to get tired so easily.

- This is too hard.

These thoughts will drive you crazy if you let them and they will certainly paralyze your progress. So how do you get over the "**buts**" and start shrinking your BUTT?

Stop making excuses. 15 minutes is better than

0. Walking is better than sitting. Drinking water is better than pop. Wherever you are is a great place to start.

Get over yourself. No one is watching you. Trust me. If you step up to the treadmill or weight bench next to me, I may look up to say hi and that's about it. I'm too busy breathing, lifting, and sweating to care about your workout and so is almost everyone else.

Realize only you carry your weight; only you can lose it. You can workout with 10 people or 10 million but at the end of the day only the calories *you* burn will contribute to your weight loss.

Understand it won't get easier. The longer you put it off the more difficult it becomes to get started.

Change SOMETHING. You may not be able to jump right in and change everything right away but you can do something right now. Changing your mind is a great place to start.

I will be honest, the "buts" I mentioned are ones that used to plague me. They may be the same for you or they may be different. The bottom line is: What are you going to do about it? How long will you allow your "buts" to keep growing your gut?

Move past your feelings and let's get to work!

Three Areas of Focus

"Diet + Exercise + Rest = Results"

~Tiffini Holmes

The three major principles to weight loss to focus on first are: eating, moving, and resting.

Before I changed my lifestyle I ate two meals a day. They were usually large; one at midday and one late night. The only moving I was doing was as part of my daily routine activity or occasionally clubbing with friends and dancing. Rest for me was non-existent. I prided myself on not needing a lot of sleep. I was the queen of thriving off 4 hours of sleep. Even now, I can't sleep more than six hours at night without feeling sluggish all day.

So let's look closer at these three things. What you are eating? How you are moving? Are you getting adequate rest? These three factors will lead to weight loss or weight gain.

You are What You Eat

When I was in graduate school for my MBA and later for my MA in psychology, I was also working fulltime. That meant, I would work all day, rush out of work to attend class at night, and arrive home around 10 pm.

Depending on how busy I was at work I would grab something quick during lunch or work straight through without eating at all. I would often pass through a drive-thru on my way to or from school. So we're talking two big meals filled with fat, preservatives, and nothing good for me.

Breaking my bad eating habits was very hard for me. My schedule didn't change and I didn't know a thing about meal prep in the beginning. So what did I do? I cut those meals in half by ordering smaller meals and I also started incorporating better "on the go" food choices like snacks! Later I cut back the number of times I ate bad meals. Then I eventually started adding more healthy food options and further decreasing the unhealthy ones.

Move It to Lose It

I don't know if anyone loves a challenge more than me. I had a fulltime, management level job, pursued an advanced degree, and began a lifestyle change all while juggling a social life, family, volunteer work, and other commitments!

In the midst of my hectic schedule I had to find time to work out. How? After having an unused, paid for, gym membership for 2-3 years I refused to buy another one. So I started walking. Each day I would get up and walk as far as I could, for as long as I could, up to an hour.

In the beginning my walk probably lasted about 20 minutes and covered about ¾ of a mile. From there, I worked my way up to longer walks 3-4 days a week, on the weekends, and on days I didn't have class. Gradually I increased to walking daily. Finally, I was ready to commit to a gym membership again, knowing this time I would actually go.

More than Beauty Rest

Finding time to rest in addition to everything else seemed somewhat impossible at first. However, it was actually easier than I originally thought it would be. With my crazy schedule, it normally took me hours to wind down at night. On less hectic days, I was usually running around like a chicken with my head cut off, trying to get everything done that had been neglected. The key for me was getting organized. Once I organized myself and my tasks it freed time up for me to rest more.

I actually began to plan my days. Friends even tease me now saying, "I started to call to see if you wanted to get together earlier but I know you stay on schedule so I didn't bother." I am really not that bad but time is so valuable to me that I make sure I spend it wisely. If I need to make several stops I map them out so I knock everything in the same area out at the same time. I also plan meals in advance and make sure I have the items I need on hand by organizing my grocery list by ingredients and location in the store.

Everything is scheduled for me now. My workouts are scheduled, I shut down each night at a designated time, I even schedule open time to make sure I rest. Planning allows me to get everything done without feeling stressed, rushed, or generally harassed. It also makes room for emergencies or contingencies not to completely derail the day or week. This allows me to fall asleep immediately and restfully.

Another important factor of rest is not just sleeping. You also have to rest your mind and spirit as well. Therefore, I now choose one day each week where I do not workout, work, or do anything other than relax.

When it comes to these three being mindful of what you eat and being active are obvious for most people. The third element, rest can be harder to grasp. Or is that just me? When I got serious about health you couldn't tell me working out seven days a week was not necessarily wise. I even remember times my trainer would suggest taking one week off every 6-8 weeks to allow my body to recover; I would be incredulous and if I am completely honest a little upset. At the time I didn't understand the importance of rest and the body needing that time to recover. Don't assume that constantly pushing yourself to or beyond the limit is best. It isn't! Adequate rest (or recovery) is a vital component along with proper diet and exercise to a healthy lifestyle.

The Workout Plan

"I hated every minute of training, but I said, 'don't

quit. Suffer now and live the rest of your life as a

champion.'" ~Muhammad Ali

I have another confession. I hate working

out. I'm not one of those people that wakes up

like, "Yes! I can't wait to get to the gym." Nope,

not me, I mean, I really don't like it at all.

However, I do it faithfully 5-6 days a week

without complaint.

A lot of people don't enjoy going to work

everyday but they do it. And do it well enough

to maintain their positions, get raises, and

receive promotions too. Working out is no

different. So, it's ok if you share the exact same

sentiment about working out with me. However, commitment outweighs feelings.

As I mentioned before, I started off walking. From walking, I graduated to a run/walk. Then I started going to the gym and got a trainer. The first two trainers I worked with had very little experience and were so unprepared for me. The first trainer, I think, was scared to work with me and probably unsure of how he could help me. The second trainer was committed to helping me as much as he knew how, but he didn't know a lot. So we would spend our sessions on the treadmill talking. Periodically he would adjust the speed or incline but that was about it. However, it was working.

I was losing a little weight but thinking I could do more than he required me to and on my own, although he was good company. So on to the next.

Like the saying goes, third time's the charm. I met yet another trainer. He was definitely not like the first two. The first words out of his mouth were, "You can do more than walk on the damn treadmill." I should have left the gym and never returned! It was the first day I began training with *Fitness Representative Personal Training*. I went in with an open-mind but nearly closed it about five minutes into our first session.

My trainer asked me to do things I had never done before, things I never thought I could do, and things I am not sure I want to do ever again. One of the very first things he asked me to do was jump up on the curb with both feet at the same time. It doesn't seem like a major feat but I am not fond of having both feet off the ground at the same time, having to clear an object, and land without injury. But I did it. He also challenged me to run. It wasn't fast but no other trainer and asked me to do so and I certainly didn't try it on my own. Plus, it wasn't just any running; he had me running in the SAND! Yet I did it and kept coming back.

I trained with him three times a week, and followed the plan he provided on my own the other three days of the week I worked out.

You know another thing I did? I lost weight. Moreover, I also lost a lot more of my fear around working out and losing weight.

Keys to a great workout:

Dynamic Warm-Up: Move while you stretch. A dynamic warm-up heats your body and muscles, increases your heart rate, and improves your range of motion. Some great moves are: jumping jacks, squats, and/or 5-10 minutes walking or a slow jog on the treadmill.

Body Weight Exercises: Push-ups, lunges, hips raises, and mountain climbers build muscle, increase your heart rate, and burn a lot of calories. These can easily be done at home and can be modified to fit any fitness level. As you get stronger you can increase the difficulty. An added benefit to body weight exercises is; most work multiple muscle groups.

Cardio: Doing cardio after weighted exercise burns more fat. Some cardio to try: walking, running, dance classes, and boot camps. If you need lower impact cardio: swimming, biking, and machines like the elliptical or rower. Cardio is important for cardiovascular health and shedding the excess fat covering those coveted six pack abs!

Stretch: Stretching after a workout is the best pain reliever I have ever met. Seriously, there is a noticeable difference the day after a workout, if

I took the time to stretch or not. It helps the muscles recover. Stretching also cools the body down gradually instead of abruptly stopping after the workout. The gradual cooling is important for the body's equilibrium. Stretching also helps prevent cramping.

Before beginning any workout program you should consult your physician and have a clear understanding of any necessary precautions. That being said, almost 100% of the time our body is capable of doing more than our mind believes we can so do your best to go beyond what you think.

The Meal Plan

"Be mindful of what you feed your mind, your body,

and your spirit." ~Tiffini Holmes

Weight loss is not all exercise. Weight loss is also about eating right to get the right results. I would even say, it's mostly about eating right.

Maybe you're not specific about the amount of weight you want to lose but more interested in losing inches off your waist. Perhaps, you aren't interested in losing weight at all and are more concerned with being healthy overall. No matter your ultimate goal, you still need to be cognizant of the foods you eat and how they impact your body.

Things like high blood pressure, high

cholesterol, and diabetes are not illnesses restricted to overweight individuals. Unhealthy eating habits at any size can lead to these and other harmful illnesses. One of the great mysteries of weight loss is to figure out how to lose pounds or inches without sacrificing the food you love to eat.

I love good food. I knew from day one that I couldn't commit to doing anything weight loss related that didn't involve good food. Which is why, for my plan initially, I didn't eliminate anything from my diet. I identified foods that I ate too much of: French fries, dinner rolls, dessert, and eating out in general. I knew from previous dieting attempts that cutting all of these things out immediately and completely wouldn't work for me. So I cut back instead.

I essentially weaned myself while simultaneously trying to add in better options. Initially, I did things like only have fries three times a week and on those days I couldn't have dessert. I would only eat out 1-2 times a week. Additionally, I would require myself to eat a fruit or vegetable with every meal.

Once I was comfortable with that, I cut back on more bad habits and added even more healthy choices. I started learning the differences between saturated and unsaturated fats, whole wheat vs. whole grain, and the value of steel cut oatmeal over instant. I became a student of food and nutrition.

I learned about using different cooking methods along with fresh herbs and spices to add flavor instead of oils and butters. I also began to study the concept of food as medicine. That is another topic for another book. Notice I haven't talked about calorie counting, macronutrients, or carb cycling. Honestly, I wasn't there yet.

That realistic component is why so many dieters tend to fail. They go jumping into an eating plan that has been said to help drop weight fast or remove stubborn belly fat without considering how sustainable it is. As a result they crash within weeks due to binge eating. Let the last time you did that be the last time you do that.

Tips for Eating Better:

Cut back until you can cut out. If you have eaten potato chips everyday for the last five years, chances are you can't stop cold turkey. Reduce the number of servings you have per week until you are down to one serving a month. Continue to cut back until they're gone forever.

Find better alternatives. Go from eating regular yogurt to Greek yogurt. Stop drinking fruit juice and start eating the whole fruit. Make sure you are making the healthiest, tastiest choices possible.

Don't skip meals. I will spare you a long lecture about missing meals and slowing down your metabolism, which burns fewer calories, which means less fat/pounds coming off. Beyond that, food is fuel. Your body runs off the energy provided by what you eat.

All food that is marketed as healthy ISN'T. Take the time to compare labels. If you look at most turkey bacon compared to center cut pork bacon or most granola bars to a cookie the nutrition facts are shockingly similar and sometimes the "healthy" choice is worse. Guard against accidental self sabotage by reading the labels.

Eat whole foods. I'm not talking about the grocery store chain. Although, there is nothing wrong with it, and there are a few products I can only get there, so I am a fan. However, what I mean is to purchase foods in their most "whole" and unprocessed states. Think about it. Processed food is preserved so that it lasts longer. Those same preservatives still work to preserve those foods in our bodies, making them harder to break down. What happens to the remaining food our bodies don't break down? It gets stored as fat.

Try new things. I was the queen of, "I don't like that," whether I had tasted it before or not. However, I knew I wouldn't last long only eating the vegetables I liked, which at the time were: broccoli, spinach, lettuce, and corn. I had to find new vegetables or new ways to prepare old vegetables.

Allow your palette to adjust. This is very bittersweet. So many things I used to love I can no longer eat because they don't taste good anymore. I am very sensitive to both salt and sugar now. That means that French fries and dessert rank much lower on my list of favorites. Heck, sometimes I even crave certain vegetables now. I told you! This is very bittersweet.

Tools You Can Use

"Knowing the path to take is easy. Actually walking it is the hard part. But the transformation along the way.... priceless! Start walking." ~Tiffini Holmes

Throughout my weight loss transformation journey, I have relied on numerous resources to help me through it. While my results directly and solely reflect my efforts, having guidance has been invaluable. I want to share with you a few of my staples and go-to resources and how they impacted my own weight loss transformation journey.

God. My weight loss transformation in progress

has been a complete faith journey. I didn't know if I could do this before and for a long time during. I prayed for strength, guidance, endurance, the will to do it, focus, you name it. Sometimes, I had to pray through a workout because it felt so tough. LOL! But really, when you face such a daunting and personal task you need something bigger than you to lean on and restore you when it seems too difficult. God sustains me daily and was especially important throughout this process.

Personal trainer. A couple chapters ago I shared my experience of finding a personal trainer. It took me some trial and error to find the right trainer but when I did, I lost 92 pounds in one year with him and kept it off. As my trainer always says and I find it to be true, "you don't push yourself as hard as a trainer will." I will go one step further and say I wouldn't have even tried certain things without a professional convincing me I could. Additionally, working with a trainer takes the guesswork out of figuring out what will work for you on your own.

Finally, it adds accountability. You are more likely to workout on your own when you know you will have to keep up with the ever-increasing intensity that working with a personal trainer requires.

Health coach. While accountability is also a

major component of coaching, a health coach is vastly different from a personal trainer. A health coach assists you with changing behavior. The focus is more on the mental and emotional components of creating a lifestyle of wellness. For example, a health coach will help you find a solution to not having time for a workout, strategize finding time to meal prep, or help you recognize an emotional issue happening every day that prompts you to eat or stress out. This is a compliment to a personal trainer. Having a health coach and personal trainer work together on a wellness plan tailored to your needs is very advantageous.

Employer benefits. Most benefit programs

include an employee assistance program. This part of the health plan gives you access to discounted gym memberships, a nutritionist, health newsletters with wellness tips, and more. There may even be weight management specialists that are covered by the insurance plan. Stop in your HR office, call the HR hotline, visit the website, or call your benefits provider to find out what type of benefits are covered under your plan.

Fitbit or other fitness-tracking device. When I first got my Fitbit I spent many a night pacing around my room at 11:30 pm desperately trying to reach my step count goal. I also, diligently looked at my stats every day to see how many calories I burned, how much sleep I got, and when I was "inactive" (took less than 250 steps in an hour). My favorite part is the challenges. Nothing makes me work harder than the friendly competition of a Work Week Hustle.

Health and fitness apps. MyFitnessPal, Couch to 5k, and Waterlogged are just a few wellness apps that are great. Whether you are tracking your water intake, counting calories, or learning to run long distance, there is an app for it and it can act as a goal assistant to help you stay on track.

Social media. Use it for encouragement,

inspiration, motivation, and accountability. Follow experts and people who have successfully done what you are trying to do or people who are currently in transformation just like you. There is nothing like knowing you aren't alone and relating to someone else's struggles. Post! Tell people what you're doing. It isn't to brag, it's to keep you accountable because now people are watching and waiting to see if you'll be consistent. Plus, your post may be just the inspiration someone else needs to get started.

Good shoes. I will be the first to admit that when I first started working out I selected my gym shoes solely based on how they matched my workout outfits. Once I realized that the wrong type of gym shoe would hurt your form, decrease your productivity, and could hurt your feet or back, I had to focus less on color coordination and more on purpose and fit. I even went to a specialty shoe store to have my gait analyzed and to be fitted for the best shoe for me and my goals.

This short list of resources is enough to get you started and to keep you going. Again, don't try to overload yourself and do too much too fast. Choose one or two and start there. Once you're used to the new additions and have some increased confidence that you're on the right track, continue to add other tools and resources that will help you stay accountable, encourage you to keep going, and help you as you go along the way. All these things are important to your total weight loss transformation journey.

A Whole New World

"We all have possibilities we don't know about.

We can do things we don't even dream we can do."

Dale Carnegie

My fitness journey began with one, attainable goal, to concur the 14 stairs from my garage to the first floor of my building without getting winded.

It was so important for me to succeed at losing weight this time around. It was the one thing in life I had failed at on multiple occasions. Even though I don't like failure, I'd allowed this to go on for too long. Mainly, because I wasn't having any health issues, I was still leading a fun and active life, and from a vanity perspective I was still cute.

Being overweight didn't impact my confidence and had no bearing on my social life. The only thing it hindered was my ability to shop anywhere I wanted for clothes. But that was enough for me. I was tired of being forced to buy clothes from a handful of plus size retailors or catalogs. I wanted more options. I wanted to get on a plane and not wonder if I would need a seatbelt extender. I used these types of measures as my milestones.

I was so excited for the day when I could shop in any store for more than just accessories.

It's funny, now I hate shopping because it means trying everything on because the sizes will vary from store to store. I also dislike buying clothes and paying a lot of money for them because I know sooner rather than later they will be too big and I will have wasted money. So now I thrift! I shop primarily at bargain, closeout, and thrift stores.

Accomplishing my weight loss goals has allowed me to do things including and beyond fitness that I may have never done before. It goes way beyond shopping where I want now. Since beginning my journey, I have taken swimming lessons, which is huge for me. Previously, I was too afraid because I had almost drowned as a child and have never forgotten that day. Things like running, playing tennis, storming the stadium (an event where you climb up and down 6000 stairs in a stadium; I did it twice) was never really even on my agenda. But every time I run a little further or faster, I feel a great sense of pride.

I left corporate America and started my own business. And the list continues. As I slowly added to my list of weight loss, diet, and fitness goals, I also added to my life goals as well. Now I try things just for fun, to test my new limits, and to challenge myself to keep improving. There were days I didn't think I could lose 15 pounds let alone 150. Now knowing that I can, I have the freedom to set even larger goals for myself. As a result, I'm seeing changes in every area of my life. I'm experiencing a whole new world of possibilities being open for me. Remember, when I started my journey I wasn't sure I could lose 200lbs. Along the way, I have discovered there is no way I can't!

That's the point of this chapter. Once you take the limits off yourself in one area, limitations in other areas with follow suit. There is a constant battle between the old me and the new me. However, I must say, the new me is kicking my old me's butt.

With some effort there is so much we can do. The more we understand the power of CAN the less we consider the possibility of can't. Here are some things you can do to remove your own limitations:

Try: At least make an attempt before deciding it can't be done.

Be Consistent: One time won't cut it. You are what you repeatedly do.

Push: Work hard to get better, and then work harder to become your best!

Know: It will take effort, but you can do it.

The Journey

"I am bigger than the limits that are put on me. It all has to do with the individual journey." Ziggy Marley

As I've shared throughout this book, losing 150 pounds on my way to my goal of 200 has been a journey. I worked out, I ate right, and I lost weight. However, I didn't escape the many pitfalls along the way.

At one point on my journey, I had started traveling for work to the point I was living in a hotel for 2 weeks at a time, home for 3 days, and then back on the road again. I gained 50 pounds back. However, I refused to let that be an excuse to fall completely off my weight loss journey.

Even though I had to work harder to lose those 50 pounds again, I haven't looked back since.

How did I lose it? How do I keep losing it? How do I make sure I don't gain?

I stay focused.

Going to the gym is a job. That means it isn't optional. There was a period of time when I was kind of obsessive about going to the gym. I was there 7 days a week. When my trainer would talk about a rest day, or heaven forbid occasionally taking a week off to rest I would scoff and say no way.

Now, while I have learned the benefit of rest periods I am still at the gym, the beach, or somewhere exercising 5-6 days a week. I get bored easily and the body needs to be shocked anyway, so I change up my workouts regularly. When the weather permits I'm outside as much as possible. I vary my cardio routines between machines like the stair-climber, elliptical, and treadmill. I also include calisthenics like jumping jacks. I used to be so intimidated by the guys in the weight area; I would try to avoid it. However, I now lift weights. Even though I am still not completely comfortable over there, I force myself to look straight ahead, do my thing, and move on.

My eating is purposeful. I'm very aware of everything I consume. I still enjoy food but I'm always thinking ahead about what I'm going to eat. I meal prep faithfully. This saves me time and excuses. No matter how late I get home there is a meal waiting because I prepared it in advance. If I wake up late, no worries, my container of oatmeal is sitting on the top shelf of the refrigerator. I just have to grab it, add a little water and pop it in the microwave when I get where I'm going.

I still enjoy the occasional meal out. But I prepare for that as well. I look at the menu in advance to decide what I'm going to eat. I keep my diet leading up to that day very clean to make allowances for going out. I allow myself a cheat meal. Notice I said meal, not day. A cheat day can potentially erase a week of your efforts. Additionally, in the quest to create healthy habits you don't want to reintroduce bad habits in large quantities on a recurring basis.

I created healthier habits. In the beginning you couldn't pay me to get on the scale to track my progress. I still don't like it to this day. Why? The scale doesn't tell the whole story. It certainly doesn't always show how hard I work or how disciplined I have been. Therefore, it can be discouraging when you know you have burned a million calories and only lost one pound. So for a while I didn't get on the scale. Instead I tracked how many days I stuck to my meal plan, how many times I went to the gym, and how my clothes fit. Consistency breeds results.

I started tracking my mile time, and how

many push-ups I could do. I still use these methods today. I measure my fitness, not my weight. I do get on the scale once a month to track my progress there also. But my primary focus is healthy living. Am I moving enough? Am I eating the right foods, at the right times? How do I feel physically, mentally, and emotionally? Am I getting stronger?

TRUTH IS: I didn't need anyone to tell me I needed to lose weight. I could look in the mirror and see it myself. I knew the health risks of obesity. I made a choice (conscious or unconscious) to be the way I was.

TRUTH IS: I tended to lie to myself more than anyone else lied to me or withheld the truth from me. The excuses I made for why I didn't or couldn't change were not true. I was raised to know I can do all things. It takes courage, hard work, and time but it can be done.

TRUTH IS: I knew the truth and chose not to acknowledge it. I can see the truth about others so clearly, so my vision didn't suddenly go bad when I looked at myself. I chose to focus on what I wanted to see or I didn't look at all.

TRUTH IS: Contrary to the infamous movie line, "You can't handle the truth." I could handle it. And in order to transform myself, I had to handle it. I had to grow to be honest with myself in all things. I had to recognize the truth; my weight was a problem. I had to be honest about the effort I wasn't making, and I had to acknowledge the ultimate truth; the only thing stopping me was me!

TRUTH IS: Knowing all these other truths, I chose to change. I chose to begin doing all the things I hadn't been doing before to get my health and life on track. I transformed my eating habits, started working out, and vowed to never go back to living the way I was before.

TRUTH IS: I don't always get it right. I still don't always get enough rest; sometimes I will get busy and forget to eat dinner. It happens. I forgive myself. I move on.

MY FINAL TRUTH IS: I will never quit trying. Every day I get up determined to be better than I was the day before.

No question, I have had a lot of help. I have an awesome trainer that provides me with workouts that challenge and encourage me, health and fitness tips that were invaluable on how to eat better, and courage to try some crazy stuff that I never would think of on my own.

My friends have encouraged me along the way. They've been willing to forgo dessert at our favorite restaurants for my sake, and are quick to compliment me, even when I know I haven't lost an ounce. Even with all the support, I would not have been successful thus far if I didn't WANT IT and wasn't wiling to GO GET IT for myself.

If you don't remember anything else from this book remember that *you* are solely responsible for your gains and losses.

Part III: Total Wellness Transformation

It's Not All About You

"Setting an example is not the main means of

influencing others, it is the only means."

~Albert Einstein

The success of your weight loss and

transformation journey is so important because

while it is mainly about you, it's not totally

about you. Someone is always watching and

your behavior has the potential to influence his

or her choices as well.

Not that any of my workouts are easy but

I remember a specific day that from the time I

stepped on the sand to begin training it was a

struggle. My trainer and I didn't do anything we

hadn't done before but for some reason after

about 10 minutes I was ready to quit.

I didn't though. I suffered in silence and did my best to push through. It wasn't pretty. It wasn't fun. I didn't even feel accomplished. I was just glad it was over. But as I was leaving, an older, overweight woman stopped me to tell me what a good job I had done and how seeing me workout inspired her.

She related a story about feeling bad early that morning after going into Starbucks and seeing some women that were much smaller in their short shorts and feeling like she could never be that size. Well, I don't know that she or my thighs or butt will ever be in a pair of daisy dukes but if seeing me sweat it out sparks her drive to live a healthier lifestyle I am with it.

To be honest, I hate it when people see me working out and think it is a big deal or some great feat. I really am no different than anyone else that works out. However, as I meet more people and hear more stories, I realize no matter what I think, people are watching and they are being motivated.

So when I workout it's not just about me. I'm doing it so that others know they can too. I can't quit because that may prompt someone else to quit.

We're not in this world by ourselves. Whether directly or indirectly, our actions impact and influence others. Always choose wisely, you never know who is watching and being inspired by you.

I don't know what the lady I met will do but I know I did my part in planting the seed. When you know better you not only do better but you educate others on how to do better as well.

Love is Honest

"Tough love may be tough to give but it is a necessity of life and assurance of positive growth."

~T.F.Hodge

I remember reading an article about a fit guy that fell in love with an overweight woman and they were living happily ever after.

As an overweight woman who has dated fit guys before, I didn't know why that article was considered newsworthy, but I digress. It was the tone of the article that concerned me. Behind the text of the article was the insinuating question, "why would the "fit guy" want to be with the "fat girl", which was ridiculous. Yet throughout the article and comments, no one seemed to address the most important issue, HEALTH.

The guy talked about how much he loved his girlfriend and that he finds her attractive. How he loves her confidence and that she has a great personality. I believed him and I thought, "That's great!" I appreciated that he was attracted to her inside and out. He also said she doesn't have to lose weight and he loved her just like she is. Problem. That is what my boyfriend's, friends, and family always told me when the subject of weight came up.

Being unhealthy mind, body, or spirit is not okay! We love people unconditionally, no question. But we are also obligated to encourage our loved ones to be their healthiest selves. So in LOVE we have to encourage them to live a healthier lifestyle. I know weight talks can be sensitive but if someone were drinking, smoking, or drugging themselves to death we wouldn't hesitate to step in. The same should be done with weight.

Also, don't be deceived by your "skinny, fat" friends. These are people who look to be a normal or acceptable weight, but also have horrible eating and exercise habits. They need to get it together too. The reality is: no one *wants* to be fat.

What can you do?

Be real. I know you love them but be honest

enough to admit they need to get their health together.

Be sensitive. Know your audience and the tone they will be most receptive to.

Be consistent. Don't encourage them to be healthy one week then make their favorite dessert the next.

Be involved. Work out with them. When you take those romantic late night beach strolls, pick up the pace and do some brisk walking intervals. Also, sex can be quite the calorie burner (or so I am told; where's my halo?)

Be patient: I wish change happened overnight but it doesn't. Give your loved one support and time to make changes.

Whether we like the truth or not it's

always easier to hear it from someone we love.

Fortunately, I have a great doctor that I have a

great relationship with that consistently told me

I needed to do something different. It took years

for me to finally listen but I am so glad I did.

Love is a lot of things but one of the most

important things is: love is HONEST!

Exercise: I Love You This Much

This is an opportunity to show some love.

Write a letter to yourself or someone you care

about. Explain:

1. What you love about them

2. What concerns you have about their

    health: mind, body, and spirit

3. What you suggest they do

4. If they want your help or who can help if

    it's a letter to yourself

5. Why their/your health is so important to

    you

The Results

"I've always believed that if you put in the work, the results will come." ~Michael Jordan

One decision to change one thing transformed my whole life. I began my journey simply wanting to lose weight. What happened instead has been priceless. I think the best way to explain is to break it out by category.

Body

- I went from a size 28 in women's plus to my current size 18 (bottom) 14/16 (tops).

- I used to take 25 minutes to walk one mile. Now I jog one mile in about 13:30 minutes.

- I could barely do 10 women's style push-ups. Now I can do 4 sets of 25 fairly easy.

- Previously you couldn't pay me to work out. Now you couldn't pay me not to.

- I refused to try certain things physically. Now, it may take me a few minutes to mentally prepare but not attempting it isn't even an option.

- My body craves vegetables. That wasn't even a goal. I guess it's a bonus!

- I've cut my caloric intake in half. At my peak weight I was consuming probably about 3200 calories a day. Now as I continue my transformation I average around 1600 per day.

Mind

- I'm confident I can do anything. Weight was the pink elephant in the room (pun intended). I knew it was there but I didn't know I could get rid of it. I can and I did. There is nothing I can't do.

- My no means no. I've learned not to compromise on my health or things that benefit me. If it's right for me, I'm going to do it no matter what anyone else says or thinks.

- I am cognizant that my life is one of my choosing. If at any time I don't like something about it, I can choose to change it.

- My weight was a symptom of the real problem(s). I didn't know how to eat and I wasn't interested in exercise. Combine that with being busy and stressed and you get weight gain. Learning to manage stress and time management was essential to my success.

- I am the cause and the cure. I was responsible for my weight gain and my weight loss. While there may have been external factors influencing my decisions, it was always only me taking action to negatively or positively impact my weight. I decided to only have a positive impact.

Spirit

- I love me and I show it. I have always loved me but oftentimes I neglected me, which resulted in weight gain. Now I stay in tune with myself and what I'm feeling. Then I deal with managing the feeling and not allowing it to change my habits.

- I'm motivated to be better. Each achievement is simply a stepping-stone to the next. I don't know what my best self entails but I am excited to strive for it every day.

- I stress less. I feel so much more in control of my life. I used to feel like I was always scrambling to keep up with my life yet usually a step or two behind. Now, I'm taking life in stride, dealing with things as the come, and not sweating the big or small stuff because I know everything will work out, as it should.

- I'm free. This is the best feeling in the world. I'm living the life of my choosing and loving it. I'm empowered and confident in my ability. I'm willing to do what is right for me with national approval or none. It's all good!

  The results above are selfishly all related to me and what I've accomplished. However, it's the external results that I am most proud of! Total Transformation Wellness Coaching was born from it. I started TTWC to help others achieve their life goals while improving their health mind, body, and spirit.

I realized losing weight is so hard because the focus is all wrong. Sure diet and exercise are essential but what about the behavior change, identifying the cause of bad habits, and working to mitigate them so that a new lifestyle is sustainable. TTWC specializes in seeing the big picture and breaking it down into manageable goals and objectives that when put together complete the puzzle for my clients. I also get the opportunity to speak and present workshops to groups, motivating them to pursue their goals with enthusiasm. Finally, through social media I have been able to reach thousands and inspire them to begin their own transformations.

Total Wellness

You may never get anyone's permission or approval to be great. Thank God you don't need it! Greatness is your destiny; be relentless, go get it.

~Tiffini Holmes

This chapter by far is the toughest to write. To attempt to articulate the mental and emotional transformation I've experienced almost leaves me speechless.

Even without yet hitting my final goal of 200 pounds lost, I feel accomplished. As I've said, the thought of losing 200 pounds was once overwhelming. It still overwhelms me and I'm almost there.

I've learned so much about myself on my

weight loss journey. I learned that I have usually chosen the easy route. Keep in mind, easy is relative. I believe this is the main reason I was unconsciously reluctant to get serious about weight loss for quite some time. I honestly didn't want to fail. I was comfortable with myself at the heavier weight so why take on a task that I might not succeed at and feel like a failure?

It's the same fear that made me reluctant to become an entrepreneur. Sure I had started a couple businesses before but they were strictly side jobs that didn't interfere with my day job, which I worked diligently and didn't plan to give up.

I decided to take the risk of failure and I went forward anyway. As I shed the body weight, I also shed the weight of only doing what was expected of me, the weight of what if, and the weight of staying inside the box.

Somewhere in the process for me and I suspect for everyone, I started to shed my self-imposed limitations. I had a great life before but it got even better. I didn't know what I was missing until I found it. Sometimes I regret that it took me so long to figure it out.

I waver about the feeling of regret. I'm not big on dwelling on the past but I think to acknowledge how things could be different demonstrates an increased level of consciousness.

All that being said there are many things I

sometimes regret about life.

- I regret I let my weight get out of control.

- I regret that I have loved ones that don't prioritize their health and well being.

- I regret that people die before they have a chance to grow old and then pass peacefully in their sleep.

- I regret that I let things beyond my control bother me.

- I regret that choices I've made have had such costly consequences.

- I regret that I sometimes give more attention to the bad things that happen and not enough to the good things.

All right, enough! It's clear I have regrets. But I also know that after the regrets come regrouping, refocusing, and finally rejoicing.

How to Move Past Your Regrets

Regroup: Think everything through, process it, organize it, and then let it go.

Refocus: Now that everything is settled in your mind, remember what your focus is and get back to doing what you do best, accomplishing goals.

Rejoice: You made it through! Despite all that has gone wrong you not only survived, you found a way to thrive.

Life is a process and I have a bad habit of only wanting to experience the good parts. But it's like planting a seed. In order for it to grow it needs sunlight, rain, soil, and good old manure. Some days we get a good dose of manure and a lot of rain. However, we must trust that we are planted in good soil and sunshine is in the forecast. It's unrealistic to think we will only be in the rejoicing phase. We must always methodically work at getting past the regret.

The reason regret is a double-edged sword is because I believe incidents in our past shape our future. If I hadn't battled the bulge I probably wouldn't be writing this book, possibly not running my own business, and certainly not helping others create their own transformation experiences. I needed to go through these things to grow. How can I regret experiences that have made me who I am today?

Sometimes I joke that my tear ducts were broken until I started my path to good health. I don't think I have ever cried so much. The tears have been a mix of happy and sad, fear and triumph, joy and pain. At times they have come in the middle of a workout when I thought I wasn't going to make it, or at the end when I did make it. Sometimes it was in euphoria over a new business idea. Other times it was when an event didn't garner as many attendees as I anticipated. Because I usually did what was easy for me, I was rarely emotionally invested enough in my endeavors to feel much of anything when it was finished. Beyond basic pride and integrity in a job well done I wasn't overly moved if it did or didn't succeed.

Today, I challenge myself daily in all

three areas: mind, body, and spirit because all three areas must be actively engaged and healthy. Weakness in one area weakens the other areas too. I know this because mentally and emotionally I was fine. I was confident, had no depression, was a goal getter, had happy, balanced relationships, and so on.

Yet, as I started to get in shape physically, I got stronger mentally and even more stable emotionally. I liken the relationship of the mind, body and spirit, to the body itself. If I sprain my right ankle, instantly my left leg starts to compensate by being the load bearing leg all the time. My abs begins to engage to provide better balance, and my right leg shifts differently to accommodate the tenderness of my right ankle.

When we are out of whack in one area, the other two pick up the slack.

For example, when you are emotionally drained you feel the physical effects, when you are mentally challenged it can make you emotionally irritable. Finally, when you have physical issues it can stress you mentally.

Good health is all encompassing. It means you have a healthy body, mind, and spirit. Anyone without ALL three in balance is unhealthy. It's easy to target the obvious (weight) and completely ignore all the other indicators of health that may be invisible to the naked eye. So what is the solution?

Mind your own health. Make sure you are

practicing a healthy lifestyle mind, body, and spirit before you start critiquing someone else's.

Focus on Total Wellness. Understand that emphasis needs to be placed on total wellness not just physical.

Get the facts. If you don't know, don't assume to know based on looks alone, go to the doctor and find out your status.

Advocate. Be concerned for everyone's total health.

Act in LOVE. This should probably be number one on the list. Because when you truly love yourself, you take care of yourself.

Final Thoughts

Be ready to work hard.

Expect positive results.

You are in control of what you do.

Only persistence will win when skill is lacking.

Unique is your journey. Don't compare it to anyone else's.

Rest when needed but don't ever quit.

Believe you can do it.

Even when it looks like you can't.

Stop doubting yourself.

Take time to appreciate your progress.

This is a great daily affirmation. I strongly encourage you to post this page on your bathroom mirror, bedroom door, your refrigerator, or as a phone or computer screensaver. Make sure it is someplace you will see it often and be reminded and encouraged to always, be your best self!

###

About the Author

Tiffini Holmes, owner of Total Transformation Wellness Coaching, is an American Council on Exercise (ACE) certified Health Coach and has more than 15 years of coaching in the human resources field. Coach Tiffini is also fully vested in seeing their success come to fruition. She believes in total wellness mind, body, and spirit. According to her, not any one without the other is enough. After being overweight most of her life Tiffini decided to take control after tipping the scale at nearly 400 lbs. To date she has lost over 150lbs. Follow Tiffini on FB, IG, and Twitter: @ttwcoach